VEGAN

AYURVEDA COOKBOOK

FOR WOMEN

PLANT BASED AYURVEDIC RECIPES TO BALANCE HORMONES, BOOST FERTILITY, REDUCE STRESS, MANAGE WEIGHT AND SUPPORT OVERALL WOMEN'S WELLNESS AND VITALITY

JUDY KELLY

Request for Review

Dear Reader,

Your opinion matters! We'd love to hear your thoughts on this cookbook. Please spare a moment to share your feedback:

1. Recipe Clarity
2. Recipe Variety
3. Cooking Experience
4. Usefulness
5. Overall Impressions

Help us enhance future editions! Share your review on Amazon

Thank you for being a part of our culinary journey!

Sincerely,
Judy Kelly

Table of Contents

Introduction

Embracing Ayurveda for Women's Wellness

Welcome to a journey of holistic well-being tailored uniquely for women through the time-honored wisdom of Ayurveda. This cookbook is an invitation to explore the synergy between plant-based nutrition and Ayurvedic principles, harmonizing the mind, body, and spirit in a way that celebrates femininity and vitality.

Ayurveda, the ancient Indian science of life, holds a profound understanding of individual constitution, recognizing that each woman is a mosaic of unique energies, rhythms, and needs. It's a system that reveres balance, emphasizing the power of nature's bounty in nurturing our health and restoring equilibrium.

In this culinary odyssey, we delve into the intricate tapestry of Ayurvedic wisdom, focusing on the specific needs of women's bodies and minds. From hormonal balance to fertility, stress reduction to weight management, digestive wellness to skin health, we've curated an array of plant-based recipes infused with the goodness of Ayurvedic insights.

Beyond just a collection of recipes, this cookbook is a testament to the art of mindful nourishment. It's an acknowledgment of the profound connection between what we eat and how we feel—recognizing food not only as sustenance but as a catalyst for transformation, healing, and rejuvenation.

As you embark on this gastronomic journey, expect more than just delectable flavors and wholesome ingredients. Anticipate an exploration of Ayurvedic herbs, spices, and principles ingeniously woven into each dish, intended not just to tantalize the taste buds but to support your well-being from within.

Whether you're seeking to restore hormonal balance, foster fertility, alleviate stress, manage weight healthily, or simply revel in the joy of vibrant health, this cookbook aims to be your trusted companion. Each recipe is crafted with care, with a deep understanding of Ayurveda's time-tested wisdom and its profound influence on women's holistic wellness.

May this book be a guiding light on your path to wellness, empowering you to embrace Ayurveda's gentle embrace, savoring every bite as a step towards radiance, balance, and vitality.

Here's to nourishing your inner goddess and honoring the wisdom of your body through the nourishment on these pages.

Understanding Ayurveda for Women's Health

In the ancient science of Ayurveda, the intricate balance between body, mind, and spirit is revered as the cornerstone of well-being. For women, this balance is a symphony of intricate energies, rhythms, and unique constitution that embodies the essence of femininity.

The Three Doshas

Central to Ayurveda's philosophy are the three doshas—Vata, Pitta, and Kapha—that govern the fundamental principles of the body. These doshas, representing different combinations of the five elements (ether, air, fire, water, and earth), influence our physical, mental, and emotional traits.

- Vata: Composed of ether and air, Vata governs movement and is associated with creativity, flexibility, and adaptability. In women, an imbalance in Vata can manifest as irregular menstrual cycles, anxiety, or dryness.
- Pitta: Formed by fire and water, Pitta embodies transformation and metabolism. It governs digestion, warmth, and intelligence. An imbalance may lead to issues like inflammation, hormonal disturbances, or emotional intensity.
- Kapha: Influenced by earth and water, Kapha embodies stability and structure. It governs stability, nourishment, and strength. In women, Kapha imbalance might lead to weight gain, lethargy, or excessive mucus production.

The Menstrual Cycle and Women's Health

Ayurveda recognizes the menstrual cycle as a vital aspect of a woman's overall health. It emphasizes the importance of regular menstrual flow as a sign of balanced doshas and reproductive health. Irregularities in the cycle may signal underlying imbalances that can be addressed through diet, lifestyle, and herbal remedies.

Nourishment According to Ayurveda
Ayurveda offers insights into food as medicine. It categorizes foods based on their taste (rasa), energy (virya), and post-digestive effect (vipaka), emphasizing a diet that balances the doshas. For women, this means embracing nourishing, seasonal foods that support hormonal balance, digestion, and vitality.

Lifestyle Practices for Women's Wellness
Beyond diet, Ayurveda promotes lifestyle practices that honor the natural rhythms of the body. From self-care rituals (dinacharya) to yoga, meditation, and stress reduction techniques, these practices nurture women's well-being, promoting inner harmony and resilience.

By embracing Ayurveda's holistic approach, women can harness its wisdom to restore balance, vitality, and radiant health. Understanding one's unique constitution and aligning with the rhythms of nature empowers women to navigate life's changes while nurturing their well-being from within.

Chapter 1: Breakfasts

1. Energizing Berry Breakfast Smoothie

Ingredients:
- 1 ripe banana
- 1 cup mixed berries (strawberries, blueberries, raspberries)
- 1 cup almond milk or any plant-based milk
- 1 tablespoon chia seeds

Instructions:
1. Peel the banana and place it in a blender.
2. Add the mixed berries into the blender.
3. Pour in the almond milk.
4. Sprinkle the chia seeds on top.
5. Blend all the ingredients until smooth.
6. Pour the smoothie into a glass and serve immediately.

2. Chia Seed Breakfast Bowl

Ingredients:
- 3 tablespoons chia seeds
- 1 cup almond milk or any plant-based milk
- 1 tablespoon maple syrup
- Sliced bananas or berries for topping

Instructions:
1. In a bowl, combine chia seeds, almond milk, and maple syrup.
2. Stir the mixture well.
3. Cover the bowl and refrigerate it for at least 2 hours or overnight.
4. Once the chia pudding is set, top it with sliced bananas or berries before serving.

3. Quinoa Breakfast Bowl

Ingredients:
- 1 cup cooked quinoa
- 1/2 cup coconut yogurt or any plant-based yogurt
- 1 tablespoon maple syrup or agave syrup
- Sliced mangoes or pineapples

Instructions:
1. In a bowl, mix the cooked quinoa, coconut yogurt, and maple syrup.
2. Stir until well combined.
3. Top the mixture with sliced mangoes or pineapples.

4. Green Goddess Smoothie

Ingredients:
- 1 cup spinach leaves
- 1/2 cup sliced cucumbers
- 1/2 cup frozen mango chunks
- 1 cup coconut water or almond milk

Instructions:
1. Add spinach leaves, sliced cucumbers, frozen mango chunks, and liquid into a blender.
2. Blend the ingredients until smooth.
3. Pour the smoothie into a glass and serve.

5. Avocado Toast

Ingredients:
- 2 slices of whole grain bread, toasted
- 1 ripe avocado
- Pinch of salt and pepper
- Optional toppings: sliced tomatoes, microgreens

Instructions:
1. Slice the ripe avocado in half and remove the pit.
2. Scoop the avocado into a bowl and mash it with a fork.
3. Spread the mashed avocado evenly onto the toasted bread slices.
4. Sprinkle a pinch of salt and pepper on top.
5. Add optional toppings like sliced tomatoes or microgreens.

6. Energy-Boosting Acai Bowl

Ingredients:
- 1 packet frozen acai
- 1/2 cup mixed berries
- 1/2 cup almond milk or any plant-based milk
- Toppings: sliced strawberries, granola, coconut flakes

Instructions:
1. Blend the frozen acai, mixed berries, and almond milk until smooth.
2. Pour the acai mixture into a bowl.
3. Top the bowl with sliced strawberries, granola, and coconut flakes.

7. Mango Turmeric Smoothie

Ingredients:
- 1 cup chopped mango
- 1/2 teaspoon turmeric powder
- 1/2 cup coconut water or almond milk
- 1 tablespoon hemp seeds

Instructions:
1. Combine chopped mango, turmeric powder, coconut water or almond milk, and hemp seeds in a blender.
2. Blend until smooth.
3. Serve the mango turmeric smoothie immediately.

8. Pumpkin Spice Oatmeal

Ingredients:
- 1/2 cup rolled oats
- 1 cup almond milk or any plant-based milk
- 1/4 cup pumpkin puree
- 1 tablespoon maple syrup
- Pumpkin pie spice mix (cinnamon, nutmeg, cloves)

Instructions:
1. In a saucepan, combine rolled oats, almond milk, pumpkin puree, and maple syrup.
2. Cook over medium heat, stirring occasionally, until the oats are cooked and the mixture thickens.
3. Sprinkle with pumpkin pie spice mix before serving.

9. Protein-Packed Tofu Scramble

Ingredients:
- 1/2 block firm tofu, crumbled
- 1/2 cup sautéed bell peppers, spinach, and onions
- 1/4 tcaspoon turmeric powder
- Pinch of salt and pepper

Instructions:
1. In a pan, sauté bell peppers, spinach, and onions until tender.
2. Add crumbled tofu to the pan and sprinkle with turmeric powder, salt, and pepper.
3. Cook until tofu is heated through and seasoned well.

10. Blueberry Breakfast Bowl

Ingredients:
- 1/2 cup cooked steel-cut oats
- Fresh blueberries

- Drizzle of maple syrup
- Optional: chopped nuts or seeds

Instructions:
1. Prepare steel-cut oats according to package instructions.
2. Top with fresh blueberries and drizzle with maple syrup.
3. Add optional nuts or seeds for extra crunch.

11. Coconut Yogurt Parfait

Ingredients:
- 1 cup coconut yogurt
- 1/2 cup granola
- Sliced strawberries or mangoes
- Drizzle of agave syrup (optional)

Instructions:
1. In a glass or bowl, layer coconut yogurt and granola.
2. Add a layer of sliced strawberries or mangoes.
3. Repeat layers. Drizzle with agave syrup if desired.

12. Pumpkin Spice Chia Pudding

Ingredients:
- 3 tablespoons chia seeds
- 1 cup almond milk or any plant-based milk
- 1/4 cup pumpkin puree
- 1 tablespoon maple syrup
- Pumpkin pie spice mix (cinnamon, nutmeg, cloves)

Instructions:
1. In a bowl, mix chia seeds, almond milk, pumpkin puree, and maple syrup.
2. Stir in a pinch of pumpkin pie spice mix.
3. Refrigerate for at least 2 hours or overnight before serving.

13. Apple Cinnamon Quinoa Bowl

Ingredients:
- 1 cup cooked quinoa
- Sliced apples
- Sprinkle of cinnamon
- Drizzle of maple syrup

Instructions:
1. In a bowl, mix cooked quinoa with sliced apples.
2. Sprinkle with cinnamon and drizzle with maple syrup.
3. Serve warm or cold.

14. Matcha Green Tea Smoothie

Ingredients:
- 1 teaspoon matcha powder
- 1 frozen banana
- 1/2 cup spinach leaves
- 1 cup almond milk or any plant-based milk

Instructions:
1. Blend matcha powder, frozen banana, spinach leaves, and almond milk until smooth.
2. Pour into a glass and enjoy.

15. Banana Walnut Pancakes

Ingredients:
- 1 ripe banana, mashed
- 1/2 cup oat flour or whole wheat flour
- 1/4 cup chopped walnuts
- 1/2 teaspoon cinnamon
- Coconut oil for cooking

Instructions:
1. In a bowl, mix mashed banana, flour, chopped walnuts, and cinnamon until well combined.
2. Heat coconut oil in a pan. Spoon pancake batter onto the pan. Cook until golden on both sides.

16. Turmeric Ginger Overnight Oats

Ingredients:
- 1/2 cup rolled oats
- 1 cup almond milk or any plant-based milk
- 1/2 teaspoon turmeric powder
- 1/2 teaspoon grated ginger
- 1 tablespoon maple syrup

Instructions:
1. In a jar or bowl, combine rolled oats, almond milk, turmeric powder, grated ginger, and maple syrup.
2. Stir well, cover, and refrigerate overnight.
3. Stir before serving. Add more milk if desired consistency is not reached.

17. Mediterranean Avocado Toast

Ingredients:
- 2 slices of whole grain bread, toasted
- Mashed avocado
- Sliced tomatoes
- Drizzle of olive oil
- Sprinkle of sea salt and black pepper

Instructions:
1. Spread mashed avocado onto the toasted bread slices.
2. Top with sliced tomatoes.
3. Drizzle with olive oil and sprinkle with sea salt and black pepper.

18. Mango Coconut Chia Pudding

Ingredients:
- 3 tablespoons chia seeds
- 1 cup coconut milk
- 1 ripe mango, diced
- Toasted coconut flakes for garnish

Instructions:
1. In a bowl or jar, mix chia seeds and coconut milk. Let it sit for 10 minutes.
2. Stir in diced mango.
3. Cover and refrigerate for at least 2 hours or until set.
4. Garnish with toasted coconut flakes before serving.

19. Vegan Breakfast Burrito

Ingredients:
- Whole grain wrap
- Scrambled tofu (seasoned with turmeric, cumin, salt)
- Sautéed bell peppers, onions, and black beans
- Salsa (optional)

Instructions:
1. Place scrambled tofu, sautéed veggies, and black beans in a whole grain wrap.
2. Roll up the wrap and serve with salsa if desired.

20. Energy-Boosting Fruit Smoothie

Ingredients:
- 1 cup mixed frozen fruits (berries, mangoes, pineapples)
- 1/2 cup orange juice
- Handful of spinach leaves
- 1 tablespoon hemp seeds or chia seeds

Instructions:
1. Blend frozen fruits, orange juice, spinach leaves, and seeds until smooth.
2. Pour into a glass and enjoy the refreshing smoothie.

Chapter 2: Lunches

1. Buddha Bowl

Ingredients:
- 1 cup cooked quinoa or brown rice
- 1 cup steamed kale or spinach
- 1 roasted sweet potato (cubed)
- 1/2 avocado (sliced)
- Tahini or olive oil for dressing

Instructions:
1. Cook quinoa or brown rice according to package instructions.
2. Steam kale or spinach until tender.
3. Roast sweet potato cubes in the oven until soft.
4. In a bowl, arrange quinoa, steamed greens, roasted sweet potato, and sliced avocado.
5. Drizzle with tahini or olive oil before serving.

2. Chickpea Salad Wraps

Ingredients:
- 1 can (15 oz) chickpeas, drained and mashed with a fork
- 1/4 cup finely chopped celery
- 1/4 cup finely chopped red onion
- 1/4 cup finely chopped bell peppers (any color)
- 2 tablespoons vegan mayonnaise or tahini
- Lettuce leaves or whole grain wraps

Instructions:
1. In a bowl, mix mashed chickpeas, celery, onion, bell peppers, and vegan mayonnaise or tahini.
2. Spoon the chickpea mixture onto lettuce leaves or wraps.
3. Roll up and serve.

3. Lentil Vegetable Soup

Ingredients:
- 1 cup cooked lentils
- 2 cups vegetable broth
- 1 cup diced carrots
- 1 cup diced celery
- 1 cup diced onions
- 2 cloves garlic (minced)
- 1 teaspoon cumin
- Salt and pepper to taste

Instructions:
1. In a pot, sauté onions, garlic, carrots, and celery until softened.
2. Add cooked lentils, vegetable broth, cumin, salt, and pepper.
3. Simmer for 20-25 minutes until vegetables are tender. Adjust seasoning if needed before serving.

4. Rainbow Salad with Citrus Dressing

Ingredients:
- Mixed salad greens
- Sliced bell peppers, cherry tomatoes, shredded carrots
- Sliced oranges or grapefruit segments
- Citrus vinaigrette dressing

Instructions:
1. Arrange mixed salad greens on a plate.
2. Top with sliced bell peppers, tomatoes, carrots, and citrus segments.
3. Drizzle with citrus vinaigrette dressing before serving.

5. Quinoa Stuffed Bell Peppers

Ingredients:
- 2 bell peppers (halved and deseeded)

- 1 cup cooked quinoa mixed with black beans, corn, and diced tomatoes
- 1 teaspoon cumin
- 1/2 teaspoon chili powder
- Vegan cheese (optional)

Instructions:
1. Preheat oven to 375°F (190°C).
2. Mix cooked quinoa, black beans, corn, diced tomatoes, cumin, and chili powder.
3. Stuff halved bell peppers with the quinoa mixture.
4. Optionally, sprinkle with vegan cheese.
5. Bake for 25-30 minutes or until peppers are tender.

6. Veggie Sushi Rolls

Ingredients:
- Nori seaweed sheets
- Cooked sushi rice
- Sliced avocado, cucumber, bell peppers, carrots
- Soy sauce and wasabi for dipping (optional)

Instructions:
1. Place a nori sheet on a bamboo sushi mat.
2. Spread cooked sushi rice evenly on the nori sheet.
3. Add sliced veggies, roll tightly, and slice into sushi rolls.
4. Serve with soy sauce and wasabi if desired.

7. Mediterranean Chickpea Salad

Ingredients:
- 1 can (15 oz) chickpeas, drained and rinsed
- 1/2 cucumber, diced
- 1 cup cherry tomatoes, halved
- 1/4 cup chopped red onion
- Chopped fresh parsley and mint

- Juice of 1 lemon
- 2 tablespoons olive oil
- Salt and pepper to taste

Instructions:
1. In a bowl, combine chickpeas, cucumber, tomatoes, onion, parsley, and mint.
2. Drizzle with lemon juice and olive oil. Season with salt and pepper. Toss gently and serve.

8. Vegan Caesar Salad

Ingredients:
- Chopped romaine lettuce
- Homemade croutons
- Vegan Caesar dressing
- Optional: capers, chopped artichoke hearts

Instructions:
1. Toss chopped romaine lettuce with croutons and vegan Caesar dressing.
2. Add optional toppings like capers or chopped artichoke hearts.

9. Eggplant and Chickpea Curry

Ingredients:
- 1 large eggplant, diced
- 1 can (15 oz) chickpeas, drained and rinsed
- 1 onion, chopped
- 2 cloves garlic, minced
- 1 can (14 oz) diced tomatoes
- 1 can (14 oz) coconut milk
- 2 teaspoons curry powder
- Salt and pepper to taste
- Fresh cilantro for garnish

Instructions:
1. In a pan, sauté onion and garlic until translucent.
2. Add diced eggplant, chickpeas, diced tomatoes, coconut milk, curry powder, salt, and pepper.
3. Simmer for 20-25 minutes until eggplant is tender. Garnish with fresh cilantro before serving.

10. Tempeh Lettuce Wraps

Ingredients:
- 1 package (8 oz) tempeh, crumbled
- 2 tablespoons soy sauce
- 1 tablespoon sesame oil
- 1 teaspoon minced ginger
- 1 teaspoon minced garlic
- Butter lettuce leaves
- Sliced scallions and shredded carrots for topping

Instructions:
1. In a pan, sauté crumbled tempeh with soy sauce, sesame oil, ginger, and garlic until cooked.
2. Spoon the tempeh mixture onto butter lettuce leaves.
3. Top with sliced scallions and shredded carrots before serving.

11. Tomato Basil Pasta

Ingredients:
- 8 oz whole grain pasta
- 3 cups cherry tomatoes, halved
- 2 cloves garlic, minced
- Handful of fresh basil leaves, chopped
- 2 tablespoons olive oil
- Salt and pepper to taste

Instructions:
1. Cook pasta according to package instructions.
2. In a pan, sauté garlic in olive oil until fragrant.
3. Add cherry tomatoes and cook until softened.
4. Toss cooked pasta with tomato mixture and fresh basil. Season with salt and pepper.

12. Black Bean and Corn Salad

Ingredients:
- 1 can (15 oz) black beans, rinsed and drained
- 1 cup corn kernels (fresh or canned)
- 1 bell pepper (any color), diced
- 1/4 cup red onion, finely chopped
- Juice of 1 lime
- 2 tablespoons chopped cilantro
- Salt and pepper to taste

Instructions:
1. In a bowl, combine black beans, corn, bell pepper, and red onion.
2. Add lime juice and chopped cilantro. Season with salt and pepper. Mix well before serving.

13. Sweet Potato and Kale Salad

Ingredients:
- 2 sweet potatoes, cubed and roasted
- 4 cups kale, stems removed and chopped
- 1/4 cup walnuts or pumpkin seeds
- Dressing: 2 tablespoons olive oil, 1 tablespoon apple cider vinegar, 1 teaspoon maple syrup

Instructions:
1. Roast sweet potato cubes in the oven until tender.
2. Massage kale leaves with dressing in a large bowl.

3. Add roasted sweet potatoes and nuts/seeds. Toss gently and serve.

14. Veggie Stir-Fry with Tofu

Ingredients:
- 1 block tofu, pressed and cubed
- Assorted vegetables (bell peppers, broccoli, carrots), sliced
- 2 tablespoons soy sauce or tamari
- 1 tablespoon sesame oil
- 2 cloves garlic, minced
- Cooked brown rice for serving

Instructions:
1. In a pan, sauté tofu cubes until golden. Set aside.
2. Stir-fry vegetables in sesame oil until crisp-tender. Add minced garlic.
3. Add cooked tofu back to the pan and toss with soy sauce.
4. Serve over brown rice.

15. Mediterranean Quinoa Salad

Ingredients:
- 1 cup cooked quinoa
- 1 cucumber, diced
- 1 cup cherry tomatoes, halved
- 1/4 cup red onion, finely chopped
- Kalamata olives, sliced
- Dressing: 2 tablespoons olive oil, 2 tablespoons lemon juice, 1 teaspoon dried oregano

Instructions:
1. In a bowl, combine cooked quinoa, cucumber, tomatoes, onion, and olives.
2. Whisk together olive oil, lemon juice, and oregano for the dressing.
3. Pour dressing over the salad and toss to combine.

16. Veggie Burger Wraps

Ingredients:
- Veggie burger patties (store-bought or homemade)
- Whole grain wraps or lettuce leaves
- Toppings: avocado slices, tomato, lettuce, pickles, mustard

Instructions:
1. Cook veggie burger patties according to package instructions.
2. Place the cooked patties onto wraps or lettuce leaves.
3. Add toppings and roll up the wraps or lettuce leaves. Serve.

17. Roasted Vegetable Couscous

Ingredients:
- 1 cup couscous, cooked
- Assorted vegetables (zucchini, bell peppers, onions), diced
- 2 tablespoons olive oil
- 1 teaspoon cumin
- 1/2 teaspoon paprika
- Fresh parsley for garnish

Instructions:
1. Toss diced vegetables with olive oil, cumin, and paprika.
2. Roast in the oven until tender and slightly browned.
3. Serve roasted vegetables over cooked couscous. Garnish with fresh parsley.

18. Avocado Tomato Basil Sandwiches

Ingredients:
- Whole grain bread slices, toasted
- Ripe avocado, mashed
- Sliced tomatoes
- Fresh basil leaves

- Salt and pepper to taste

Instructions:
1. Spread mashed avocado on toasted bread slices.
2. Layer with sliced tomatoes and fresh basil leaves.
3. Season with salt and pepper. Top with another bread slice to make a sandwich.

19. Spinach and Chickpea Curry

Ingredients:
- 1 can (15 oz) chickpeas, drained
- 2 cups spinach leaves
- 1 onion, finely chopped
- 2 cloves garlic, minced
- 1 teaspoon curry powder
- 1/2 teaspoon turmeric
- 1 can (14 oz) coconut milk
- Salt and pepper to taste

Instructions:
1. Sauté onion and garlic until softened.
2. Add chickpeas, spinach, curry powder, turmeric, and coconut milk.
3. Simmer for 10-15 minutes. Season with salt and pepper.

20. Vegan Tofu Caesar Salad

Ingredients:
- 1 block tofu, pressed and cubed
- Chopped romaine lettuce
- Homemade croutons
- Vegan Caesar dressing

Instructions:
1. Sauté tofu cubes until golden.

2. Toss romaine lettuce with croutons and vegan Caesar dressing.

3. Top with sautéed tofu cubes before serving.

Chapter 3: Dinner

1. One-Pot Lentil Soup

Ingredients:
- 1 cup dried lentils
- 4 cups vegetable broth
- 1 onion, diced
- 2 carrots, chopped
- 2 celery stalks, chopped
- 2 cloves garlic, minced
- 1 teaspoon turmeric
- 1 teaspoon cumin
- Salt and pepper to taste
- Fresh parsley for garnish

Instructions:
1. In a pot, sauté onion, carrots, celery, and garlic until softened.
2. Add lentils, vegetable broth, turmeric, cumin, salt, and pepper.
3. Simmer for 20-25 minutes until lentils are tender.
4. Garnish with fresh parsley before serving.

2. Chickpea and Vegetable Stir-Fry

Ingredients:
- 1 can (15 oz) chickpeas, drained
- Assorted vegetables (bell peppers, broccoli, snap peas)
- 2 tablespoons soy sauce or tamari
- 1 tablespoon maple syrup
- 1 tablespoon sesame oil
- Minced ginger and garlic
- Cooked brown rice or quinoa for serving

Instructions:
1. Sauté vegetables in sesame oil until tender-crisp.

2. Add chickpeas, minced ginger, and garlic.
3. Stir in soy sauce and maple syrup. Cook until heated through.
4. Serve over brown rice or quinoa.

3. Stuffed Bell Peppers

Ingredients:
- 4 bell peppers, halved and deseeded
- 1 cup cooked quinoa or rice
- 1 can (15 oz) black beans, drained and rinsed
- 1 cup diced tomatoes
- 1 teaspoon chili powder
- 1 teaspoon cumin
- Vegan cheese (optional)
- Fresh cilantro for garnish

Instructions:
1. Preheat oven to 375°F (190°C).
2. In a bowl, mix cooked quinoa, black beans, diced tomatoes, chili powder, and cumin.
3. Stuff bell pepper halves with the mixture.
4. Optionally, sprinkle with vegan cheese.
5. Bake for 25-30 minutes until peppers are tender.
6. Garnish with fresh cilantro before serving.

4. Coconut Curry Tofu

Ingredients:
- 1 block tofu, pressed and cubed
- 1 can (14 oz) coconut milk
- 2 tablespoons curry powder
- 1 onion, diced
- 2 cloves garlic, minced
- 1 teaspoon grated ginger
- Assorted vegetables (bell peppers, broccoli, carrots)

- Fresh cilantro for garnish
- Cooked rice for serving

Instructions:
1. Sauté onion, garlic, and ginger until fragrant.
2. Add cubed tofu and curry powder. Cook until tofu is golden.
3. Stir in coconut milk and vegetables. Simmer until vegetables are tender.
4. Garnish with fresh cilantro and serve over rice.

5. Roasted Veggie Quinoa Bowl

Ingredients:
- 1 cup cooked quinoa
- Assorted vegetables (zucchini, cherry tomatoes, red onion)
- 2 tablespoons olive oil
- 1 teaspoon dried thyme
- Salt and pepper to taste
- Lemon wedges for serving

Instructions:
1. Preheat oven to 400°F (200°C).
2. Toss vegetables with olive oil, thyme, salt, and pepper.
3. Roast in the oven for 20-25 minutes until tender and slightly browned.
4. Serve over cooked quinoa with a squeeze of lemon.

6. Spaghetti with Vegan Bolognese

Ingredients:
- 8 oz whole grain spaghetti
- 1 can (15 oz) lentils, drained and rinsed
- 1 can (14 oz) diced tomatoes
- 1 onion, diced
- 2 cloves garlic, minced
- 2 tablespoons tomato paste
- Italian seasoning, salt, and pepper to taste

- Fresh basil for garnish

Instructions:
1. Cook spaghetti according to package instructions.
2. Sauté onion and garlic until softened.
3. Add lentils, diced tomatoes, tomato paste, and seasoning. Simmer for 10-15 minutes.
4. Serve over cooked spaghetti. Garnish with fresh basil.

7. Vegan Tofu Pad Thai

Ingredients:
- 8 oz rice noodles
- 1 block tofu, pressed and sliced
- Assorted vegetables (bell peppers, bean sprouts, carrots)
- 2 tablespoons soy sauce or tamari
- 1 tablespoon maple syrup
- 1 tablespoon lime juice
- Crushed peanuts for garnish

Instructions:
1. Cook rice noodles according to package instructions.
2. Sauté tofu and vegetables until tender.
3. In a bowl, mix soy sauce, maple syrup, and lime juice.
4. Toss cooked noodles with tofu, veggies, and sauce. Serve with crushed peanuts on top.

8. Baked Falafel with Tahini Sauce

Ingredients:
- 1 can (15 oz) chickpeas, drained and rinsed
- 1/4 cup chopped parsley
- 2 cloves garlic, minced
- 1 teaspoon cumin
- 1 teaspoon coriander

- Salt and pepper to taste
- Tahini sauce for serving

Instructions:
1. Preheat oven to 375°F (190°C).
2. In a food processor, blend chickpeas, parsley, garlic, spices, salt, and pepper until a dough forms.
3. Shape the dough into small patties and place on a baking sheet.
4. Bake for 20-25 minutes until falafel is golden brown.
5. Serve with tahini sauce.

9. Mushroom and Spinach Risotto

Ingredients:
- 1 cup Arborio rice
- 4 cups vegetable broth
- 1 onion, diced
- 2 cups sliced mushrooms
- 2 cups fresh spinach
- 1/4 cup nutritional yeast (optional for cheesy flavor)
- Salt and pepper to taste

Instructions:
1. In a pot, sauté onion and mushrooms until softened.
2. Add Arborio rice and cook for a few minutes.
3. Gradually add vegetable broth, stirring occasionally until absorbed.
4. Stir in spinach and nutritional yeast. Cook until spinach is wilted.
5. Season with salt and pepper before serving.

10. Vegan Tikka Masala

Ingredients:
- 1 block tofu, pressed and cubed
- 1 can (14 oz) diced tomatoes
- 1 onion, diced

- 2 cloves garlic, minced
- 1 teaspoon grated ginger
- 1 tablespoon garam masala
- 1 teaspoon turmeric
- 1 can (14 oz) coconut milk
- Fresh cilantro for garnish
- Cooked basmati rice for serving

Instructions:
1. Sauté onion, garlic, and ginger until fragrant.
2. Add tofu, diced tomatoes, garam masala, and turmeric. Cook until tofu is golden.
3. Pour in coconut milk and simmer for 15-20 minutes.
4. Garnish with fresh cilantro and serve over basmati rice.

11. Quinoa and Vegetable Stuffed Bell Peppers

Ingredients:
- 4 bell peppers, halved and deseeded
- 1 cup cooked quinoa
- 1 can (15 oz) black beans, drained and rinsed
- 1 cup diced tomatoes
- 1 teaspoon chili powder
- 1 teaspoon cumin
- Vegan cheese (optional)
- Fresh cilantro for garnish

Instructions:
1. Preheat oven to 375°F (190°C).
2. Mix cooked quinoa, black beans, diced tomatoes, chili powder, and cumin in a bowl.
3. Stuff bell pepper halves with the mixture.
4. Optionally, sprinkle with vegan cheese.
5. Bake for 25-30 minutes until peppers are tender.
6. Garnish with fresh cilantro before serving.

12. Lentil and Vegetable Curry

Ingredients:
- 1 cup dried lentils
- 4 cups vegetable broth
- 1 onion, diced
- 2 carrots, chopped
- 2 potatoes, diced
- 2 cloves garlic, minced
- 1 tablespoon curry powder
- 1 teaspoon turmeric
- Salt and pepper to taste
- Fresh cilantro for garnish

Instructions:
1. In a pot, sauté onion, carrots, potatoes, and garlic until softened.
2. Add lentils, vegetable broth, curry powder, turmeric, salt, and pepper.
3. Simmer for 20-25 minutes until lentils are tender.
4. Garnish with fresh cilantro before serving.

13. Veggie Tofu Stir-Fry with Brown Rice

Ingredients:
- 1 block tofu, pressed and cubed
- Assorted vegetables (broccoli, bell peppers, snap peas)
- 2 tablespoons soy sauce or tamari
- 1 tablespoon maple syrup
- 1 tablespoon sesame oil
- Minced ginger and garlic
- Cooked brown rice for serving

Instructions:
1. Sauté tofu and vegetables in sesame oil until tender-crisp.
2. In a bowl, mix soy sauce, maple syrup, ginger, and garlic.
3. Pour the sauce over the tofu and vegetables. Cook until heated through.

4. Serve over cooked brown rice.

14. Vegan Coconut Curry with Chickpeas

Ingredients:
- 2 cans (15 oz each) chickpeas, drained and rinsed
- 1 onion, diced
- 3 cloves garlic, minced
- 1 can (14 oz) coconut milk
- 1 can (14 oz) diced tomatoes
- 2 tablespoons curry powder
- 1 teaspoon turmeric
- Salt and pepper to taste
- Fresh cilantro for garnish
- Cooked basmati rice for serving

Instructions:
1. Sauté onion and garlic until translucent.
2. Add chickpeas, coconut milk, diced tomatoes, curry powder, turmeric, salt, and pepper.
3. Simmer for 20-25 minutes until flavors meld.
4. Garnish with fresh cilantro and serve over basmati rice.

15. Vegan Shepherd's Pie

Ingredients:
- 4 large potatoes, peeled and diced
- 1 cup green lentils, cooked
- Assorted vegetables (carrots, peas, corn)
- 1 onion, diced
- 2 cloves garlic, minced
- 1 tablespoon tomato paste
- 1 tablespoon soy sauce or tamari
- 1 tablespoon olive oil
- Salt and pepper to taste

Instructions:
1. Boil potatoes until tender. Mash with a little olive oil, salt, and pepper.
2. Sauté onion, garlic, and vegetables until tender.
3. Add cooked lentils, tomato paste, and soy sauce. Cook for a few more minutes.
4. Transfer the lentil and vegetable mixture to a baking dish.
5. Spread mashed potatoes on top.
6. Bake at 375°F (190°C) for 25-30 minutes until the top is golden brown.

16. Vegan Pasta Primavera

Ingredients:
- 8 oz whole grain pasta
- Assorted vegetables (zucchini, bell peppers, cherry tomatoes)
- 2 tablespoons olive oil
- 3 cloves garlic, minced
- 1/4 cup vegetable broth
- Fresh basil for garnish
- Salt and pepper to taste

Instructions:
1. Cook pasta according to package instructions.
2. Sauté vegetables and garlic in olive oil until tender.
3. Add vegetable broth and cooked pasta to the pan.
4. Toss everything together until heated through.
5. Garnish with fresh basil before serving.

17. Vegan Ratatouille

Ingredients:
- 1 eggplant, sliced
- 2 zucchinis, sliced
- 2 bell peppers, sliced
- 3 tomatoes, sliced
- 1 onion, thinly sliced

- 3 cloves garlic, minced
- 2 tablespoons olive oil
- 1 tablespoon fresh thyme leaves
- Salt and pepper to taste

Instructions:
1. Preheat oven to 375°F (190°C).
2. Arrange sliced vegetables in an overlapping pattern in a baking dish.
3. Drizzle with olive oil and sprinkle with garlic, thyme, salt, and pepper.
4. Cover with foil and bake for 30 minutes. Remove foil and bake for an additional 15-20 minutes until veggies are tender and slightly caramelized.

18. Vegan Jambalaya

Ingredients:
- 1 cup brown rice
- 1 can (15 oz) kidney beans, drained and rinsed
- 1 onion, diced
- 2 bell peppers, diced
- 2 celery stalks, diced
- 3 cloves garlic, minced
- 1 can (14 oz) diced tomatoes
- 2 cups vegetable broth
- 1 teaspoon paprika
- 1 teaspoon thyme
- 1/2 teaspoon cayenne pepper (optional)
- Salt and pepper to taste

Instructions:
1. In a pot, sauté onion, bell peppers, celery, and garlic until softened.
2. Add rice, kidney beans, diced tomatoes, vegetable broth, and spices. Stir well.
3. Bring to a boil, then reduce heat, cover, and simmer for 40-45 minutes until rice is cooked and liquid is absorbed.

19. Vegan Mushroom Risotto

Ingredients:
- 1 cup Arborio rice
- 4 cups vegetable broth
- 2 tablespoons olive oil
- 1 onion, finely chopped
- 2 cups sliced mushrooms
- 1/4 cup nutritional yeast (optional)
- Salt and pepper to taste
- Fresh parsley for garnish

Instructions:
1. In a pot, heat vegetable broth and keep it warm.
2. In another pot, sauté onion in olive oil until translucent.
3. Add sliced mushrooms and cook until tender.
4. Stir in Arborio rice and cook for a few minutes.
5. Gradually add warm vegetable broth, stirring continuously until absorbed.
6. Stir in nutritional yeast, salt, and pepper.
7. Garnish with fresh parsley before serving.

20. Vegan Stuffed Butternut Squash

Ingredients:
- 2 small butternut squashes, halved and deseeded
- 1 cup quinoa, cooked
- 1 can (15 oz) black beans, drained and rinsed
- 1 cup diced tomatoes
- 1 teaspoon cumin
- 1 teaspoon chili powder
- Fresh cilantro for garnish

Instructions:
1. Preheat oven to 375°F (190°C).

2. Place butternut squash halves on a baking sheet, cut side down. Bake for 30-35 minutes until tender.
3. In a bowl, mix cooked quinoa, black beans, diced tomatoes, cumin, and chili powder.
4. Fill each butternut squash half with the quinoa mixture.
5. Bake for an additional 15-20 minutes.
6. Garnish with fresh cilantro before serving.

Chapter 4: Desserts

1. Vegan Chocolate Avocado Mousse

Ingredients:
- 2 ripe avocados
- 1/4 cup cocoa powder
- 1/4 cup maple syrup or agave nectar
- 1 teaspoon vanilla extract
- Pinch of salt
- Fresh berries for topping (optional)

Instructions:
1. Blend avocados, cocoa powder, maple syrup, vanilla extract, and salt until smooth.
2. Refrigerate for 30 minutes before serving.
3. Garnish with fresh berries if desired.

2. Vegan Banana Nice Cream

Ingredients:
- 4 ripe bananas, sliced and frozen
- 1/4 cup plant-based milk (if needed)
- Toppings: chopped nuts, shredded coconut, or cacao nibs

Instructions:
1. Blend frozen bananas until creamy. Add plant-based milk if necessary.
2. Serve immediately topped with nuts, coconut, or cacao nibs.

3. Vegan Almond Date Balls

Ingredients:
- 1 cup dates, pitted
- 1 cup almonds
- 2 tablespoons almond butter

- 1/4 teaspoon cinnamon
- Shredded coconut for coating (optional)

Instructions:
1. Blend dates, almonds, almond butter, and cinnamon in a food processor until a dough forms.
2. Roll the mixture into small balls. Optionally, roll in shredded coconut.
3. Refrigerate before serving.

4. Vegan Chia Seed Pudding

Ingredients:
- 1/4 cup chia seeds
- 1 cup plant-based milk
- 1 tablespoon maple syrup or agave nectar
- 1/2 teaspoon vanilla extract
- Fresh fruit for topping

Instructions:
1. Mix chia seeds, plant-based milk, maple syrup, and vanilla extract in a bowl.
2. Refrigerate for at least 2 hours or overnight until thickened.
3. Serve topped with fresh fruit.

5. Vegan Apple Crisp

Ingredients:
- 4-5 apples, peeled and sliced
- 1 cup rolled oats
- 1/2 cup almond flour
- 1/4 cup maple syrup
- 2 tablespoons coconut oil
- 1 teaspoon cinnamon
- Pinch of nutmeg

Instructions:
1. Preheat oven to 350°F (175°C).
2. Place sliced apples in a baking dish.
3. In a bowl, mix oats, almond flour, maple syrup, coconut oil, cinnamon, and nutmeg.
4. Sprinkle the oat mixture over the apples.
5. Bake for 30-35 minutes until golden and bubbly.

6. Vegan Coconut Mango Rice Pudding

Ingredients:
- 1 cup cooked rice
- 1 can (14 oz) coconut milk
- 1 ripe mango, diced
- 1/4 cup maple syrup or agave nectar
- 1/2 teaspoon cardamom
- Chopped nuts for topping

Instructions:
1. In a saucepan, heat coconut milk, cooked rice, maple syrup, and cardamom.
2. Simmer for 15-20 minutes until thickened.
3. Stir in diced mango.
4. Serve warm or chilled, topped with chopped nuts.

7. Vegan Pumpkin Spice Muffins

Ingredients:
- 1 3/4 cups whole wheat flour
- 1 cup pumpkin puree
- 1/2 cup maple syrup
- 1/4 cup melted coconut oil
- 1 teaspoon baking soda
- 1 teaspoon cinnamon
- 1/2 teaspoon nutmeg

- 1/4 teaspoon cloves
- Pinch of salt

Instructions:
1. Preheat oven to 350°F (175°C). Line muffin tin with liners.
2. Mix flour, pumpkin puree, maple syrup, coconut oil, baking soda, spices, and salt in a bowl until combined.
3. Divide the batter into muffin cups.
4. Bake for 20-25 minutes or until a toothpick inserted comes out clean.

8. Vegan Berry Parfait

Ingredients:
- Mixed berries (strawberries, blueberries, raspberries)
- Dairy-free yogurt or coconut cream
- Granola or crushed nuts

Instructions:
1. Layer dairy-free yogurt or coconut cream, mixed berries, and granola or crushed nuts in serving glasses.
2. Repeat layers as desired.
3. Serve immediately.

9. Vegan Chocolate Bark

Ingredients:
- 1 cup dairy-free chocolate chips
- Assorted toppings (chopped nuts, dried fruit, coconut flakes)

Instructions:
1. Melt chocolate chips in a microwave-safe bowl in 30-second intervals, stirring in between until smooth.
2. Spread melted chocolate onto a parchment-lined baking sheet.
3. Sprinkle with assorted toppings.
4. Refrigerate until firm, then break into pieces.

10. Vegan Lemon Coconut Bliss Balls

Ingredients:
- 1 cup shredded coconut
- 1/2 cup cashews
- Zest and juice of 1 lemon
- 1/4 cup maple syrup
- Extra shredded coconut for rolling

Instructions:
1. Blend shredded coconut, cashews, lemon zest, lemon juice, and maple syrup in a food processor until a dough forms.
2. Roll the mixture into small balls and coat with shredded coconut.
3. Refrigerate before serving.

These vegan Ayurvedic dessert recipes offer a delightful way to end a meal, with a variety of flavors and textures. Enjoy creating these sweet treats!Certainly! Here are ten more vegan Ayurvedic dessert recipes to complete the list:

11. Vegan Coconut Rice Pudding

Ingredients:
- 1 cup jasmine rice
- 2 cups coconut milk
- 1/4 cup maple syrup or agave nectar
- 1 teaspoon vanilla extract
- 1/2 teaspoon ground cardamom
- Sliced almonds for garnish

Instructions:
1. Cook jasmine rice according to package instructions.
2. In a saucepan, combine cooked rice, coconut milk, maple syrup, vanilla extract, and cardamom.
3. Simmer over low heat, stirring occasionally, until the mixture thickens.

4. Serve warm or chilled, garnished with sliced almonds.

12. Vegan Carrot Halwa (Gajar ka Halwa)

Ingredients:
- 4 cups grated carrots
- 2 cups almond milk
- 1/2 cup chopped dates or raisins
- 1/4 cup crushed cashews or almonds
- 1/4 cup maple syrup or agave nectar
- 1/2 teaspoon ground cardamom
- 2 tablespoons coconut oil

Instructions:
1. Heat coconut oil in a pan, add grated carrots, and sauté for a few minutes.
2. Pour almond milk and simmer on low heat until carrots are cooked and most of the liquid evaporates.
3. Add chopped dates or raisins, crushed cashews or almonds, maple syrup, and ground cardamom.
4. Cook for an additional 5-7 minutes until the mixture thickens.
5. Serve warm.

13. Vegan Chocolate Chip Cookies

Ingredients:
- 2 cups almond flour
- 1/4 cup coconut oil, melted
- 1/4 cup maple syrup or agave nectar
- 1 teaspoon vanilla extract
- 1/2 teaspoon baking soda
- 1/4 teaspoon salt
- 1/2 cup dairy-free chocolate chips

Instructions:
1. Preheat oven to 350°F (175°C). Line a baking sheet with parchment paper.
2. In a bowl, mix almond flour, melted coconut oil, maple syrup, vanilla extract, baking soda, and salt until well combined.
3. Fold in dairy-free chocolate chips.
4. Scoop spoonfuls of dough onto the baking sheet and flatten slightly.
5. Bake for 10-12 minutes until golden brown. Let cool before serving.

14. Vegan Mango Sorbet

Ingredients:
- 3 ripe mangoes, peeled and cubed
- 1/4 cup maple syrup or agave nectar
- 2 tablespoons lime juice
- Fresh mint leaves for garnish

Instructions:
1. Place cubed mangoes in a blender or food processor.
2. Add maple syrup or agave nectar and lime juice. Blend until smooth.
3. Pour the mixture into a shallow dish and freeze for at least 4 hours, stirring every hour to break up crystals.
4. Scoop and serve garnished with fresh mint leaves.

15. Vegan Date and Walnut Bars

Ingredients:
- 1 cup dates, pitted
- 1 cup walnuts
- 1/4 cup shredded coconut
- 1 tablespoon cocoa powder
- Pinch of salt

Instructions:
1. Blend dates, walnuts, shredded coconut, cocoa powder, and salt in a food processor until a sticky dough forms.
2. Press the mixture into a lined baking dish and refrigerate for at least 1 hour.
3. Cut into bars before serving.

16. Vegan Lemon Poppy Seed Muffins

Ingredients:
- 2 cups whole wheat flour
- 1/2 cup maple syrup or agave nectar
- 3/4 cup almond milk
- 1/4 cup coconut oil, melted
- Juice and zest of 2 lemons
- 2 tablespoons poppy seeds
- 1 teaspoon baking powder
- 1/2 teaspoon baking soda
- 1/4 teaspoon salt

Instructions:
1. Preheat oven to 350°F (175°C). Line a muffin tin with liners.
2. In a bowl, mix whole wheat flour, maple syrup, almond milk, melted coconut oil, lemon juice and zest, poppy seeds, baking powder, baking soda, and salt until combined.
3. Pour batter into muffin cups.
4. Bake for 18-20 minutes or until a toothpick inserted comes out clean.

17. Vegan Pistachio Rose Water Cookies

Ingredients:
- 2 cups almond flour
- 1/2 cup pistachios, chopped
- 1/4 cup maple syrup or agave nectar
- 2 tablespoons coconut oil, melted

- 1 tablespoon rose water
- 1/4 teaspoon cardamom
- Pinch of salt

Instructions:
1. Preheat oven to 350°F (175°C). Line a baking sheet with parchment paper.
2. In a bowl, mix almond flour, chopped pistachios, maple syrup, melted coconut oil, rose water, cardamom, and salt until dough forms.
3. Roll dough into small balls and place on the baking sheet. Flatten slightly with a fork.
4. Bake for 12-15 minutes until lightly golden. Let cool before serving.

18. Vegan Berry Crumble

Ingredients:
- 3 cups mixed berries (strawberries, blueberries, raspberries)
- 1 cup rolled oats
- 1/2 cup almond flour
- 1/4 cup maple syrup or agave nectar
- 1/4 cup coconut oil, melted
- 1 teaspoon cinnamon

Instructions:
1. Preheat oven to 350°F (175°C). Grease a baking dish.
2. Spread mixed berries evenly in the baking dish.
3. In a bowl, mix rolled oats, almond flour, maple syrup, melted coconut oil, and cinnamon until crumbly.
4. Sprinkle the crumble mixture over the berries.
5. Bake for 25-30 minutes until the topping is golden brown and the berries are bubbling.
6. Serve warm.

19. Vegan Coconut Mango Mousse

Ingredients:
- 2 ripe mangoes, peeled and cubed
- 1 can (14 oz) coconut milk, chilled
- 1/4 cup maple syrup or agave nectar
- 1 tablespoon lime juice
- Toasted coconut flakes for garnish

Instructions:
1. Blend cubed mangoes, chilled coconut milk, maple syrup, and lime juice in a blender until smooth.
2. Refrigerate for at least 2 hours until set.
3. Serve chilled, garnished with toasted coconut flakes.

20. Vegan Pineapple Upside-Down Cake

Ingredients:
- 1 1/2 cups whole wheat flour
- 1 cup pineapple chunks (fresh or canned)
- 1/2 cup maple syrup or agave nectar
- 1/4 cup coconut oil, melted
- 1 teaspoon baking powder
- 1/2 teaspoon vanilla extract
- Pinch of salt
- Maraschino cherries for topping

Instructions:
1. Preheat oven to 350°F (175°C). Grease a cake pan.
2. Arrange pineapple chunks in the bottom of the cake pan. Place cherries in the center of each pineapple ring.
3. In a bowl, mix whole wheat flour, maple syrup, melted coconut oil, baking powder, vanilla extract, and salt until combined.
4. Pour batter over the pineapple in the cake pan.

5. Bake for 30-35 minutes until golden brown and a toothpick inserted comes out clean.

6. Allow to cool slightly before inverting onto a plate.

Chapter 5: Snacks and Appetizers

1. Vegan Hummus with Veggie Sticks

Ingredients:
- 1 can (15 oz) chickpeas, drained
- 2 tablespoons tahini
- 2 tablespoons olive oil
- Juice of 1 lemon
- 2 cloves garlic, minced
- Salt and pepper to taste
- Assorted vegetable sticks (carrots, cucumbers, bell peppers) for dipping

Instructions:
1. Blend chickpeas, tahini, olive oil, lemon juice, garlic, salt, and pepper in a food processor until smooth.
2. Serve hummus with vegetable sticks for dipping.

2. Vegan Guacamole with Whole Grain Chips

Ingredients:
- 2 ripe avocados
- 1 tomato, diced
- 1/4 cup red onion, finely chopped
- Juice of 1 lime
- 2 tablespoons fresh cilantro, chopped
- Salt and pepper to taste
- Whole grain tortilla chips for serving

Instructions:
1. Mash avocados in a bowl.
2. Add diced tomato, chopped red onion, lime juice, cilantro, salt, and pepper. Mix well.
3. Serve guacamole with whole grain tortilla chips.

3. Vegan Sweet Potato Bites

Ingredients:
- 2 sweet potatoes, sliced into rounds
- 2 tablespoons olive oil
- 1 teaspoon smoked paprika
- 1/2 teaspoon garlic powder
- Salt and pepper to taste

Instructions:
1. Preheat oven to 400°F (200°C).
2. Toss sweet potato rounds with olive oil, smoked paprika, garlic powder, salt, and pepper.
3. Place on a baking sheet and bake for 20-25 minutes until tender.
4. Serve as a nutritious finger food.

4. Vegan Stuffed Mini Peppers

Ingredients:
- Mini bell peppers, halved and deseeded
- Vegan cream cheese
- Chopped fresh herbs (such as parsley or chives)
- Optional: diced olives or sun-dried tomatoes

Instructions:
1. Fill mini pepper halves with vegan cream cheese.
2. Sprinkle with chopped herbs and optional diced olives or sun-dried tomatoes.
3. Serve as bite-sized stuffed peppers.

5. Vegan Cucumber Avocado Rolls

Ingredients:
- 1 cucumber
- 1 ripe avocado
- Juice of 1/2 lime
- Salt and pepper to taste
- Optional: sesame seeds or chopped nuts for topping

Instructions:
1. Use a vegetable peeler to create long, thin cucumber slices.
2. Mash avocado with lime juice, salt, and pepper.
3. Spread avocado mixture onto cucumber slices and roll them up.
4. Sprinkle with sesame seeds or chopped nuts if desired.

6. Vegan Lentil and Vegetable Samosas

Ingredients:
- Samosa pastry sheets or filo dough
- 1 cup cooked lentils
- Assorted vegetables (peas, carrots, potatoes), diced and cooked
- 1 teaspoon curry powder
- Salt and pepper to taste
- Oil for brushing

Instructions:
1. Mix cooked lentils, cooked vegetables, curry powder, salt, and pepper in a bowl.
2. Cut pastry sheets into squares or rectangles.
3. Place a spoonful of the lentil and vegetable mixture in the center of each pastry piece.
4. Fold the pastry over the filling to form triangles and seal the edges.
5. Brush the samosas with oil and bake in a preheated oven at 375°F (190°C) until golden brown.

7. Vegan Roasted Chickpeas

Ingredients:
- 1 can (15 oz) chickpeas, drained and rinsed
- 1 tablespoon olive oil
- 1 teaspoon smoked paprika
- 1/2 teaspoon cumin
- 1/2 teaspoon garlic powder
- Salt and pepper to taste

Instructions:
1. Preheat oven to 400°F (200°C).
2. Pat chickpeas dry and toss them in a bowl with olive oil, smoked paprika, cumin, garlic powder, salt, and pepper.
3. Spread chickpeas on a baking sheet and roast for 25-30 minutes until crispy.

8. Vegan Spinach Artichoke Dip

Ingredients:
- 1 can (14 oz) artichoke hearts, drained and chopped
- 2 cups fresh spinach, chopped
- 1 cup raw cashews, soaked and drained
- 1/4 cup nutritional yeast
- 2 cloves garlic, minced
- Juice of 1 lemon
- Salt and pepper to taste
- Whole grain crackers or vegetable sticks for dipping

Instructions:
1. Blend soaked cashews, nutritional yeast, garlic, lemon juice, salt, and pepper with a little water until smooth to make cashew cream.
2. Mix chopped artichoke hearts, chopped spinach, and cashew cream in a bowl.
3. Serve with whole grain crackers or vegetable sticks.

9. Vegan Sushi Rolls with Quinoa

Ingredients:
- Nori seaweed sheets
- Cooked quinoa
- Assorted vegetables (cucumber, avocado, carrot sticks)
- Soy sauce or tamari
- Pickled ginger and wasabi (optional)

Instructions:
1. Place a nori sheet on a bamboo sushi mat.
2. Spread a thin layer of cooked quinoa over the nori sheet.
3. Arrange assorted vegetables along the bottom edge of the nori sheet.
4. Roll the nori tightly and slice into sushi rolls.
5. Serve with soy sauce or tamari, pickled ginger, and wasabi if desired.

10. Vegan Buffalo Cauliflower Bites

Ingredients:
- 1 head cauliflower, cut into florets
- 1/2 cup almond flour
- 1/2 cup almond milk
- 1 teaspoon garlic powder
- 1 teaspoon onion powder
- 1/2 cup buffalo sauce
- Vegan ranch or blue cheese dressing for dipping

Instructions:
1. Preheat oven to 450°F (230°C). Line a baking sheet with parchment paper.
2. Mix almond flour, almond milk, garlic powder, and onion powder in a bowl to create a batter.
3. Dip cauliflower florets into the batter, then place them on the baking sheet.
4. Bake for 20 minutes, flipping halfway through.

5. Toss the baked cauliflower in buffalo sauce.
6. Serve with vegan ranch or blue cheese dressing for dipping.

11. Vegan Mediterranean Stuffed Grape Leaves

Ingredients:
- Grape leaves (canned or fresh)
- 1 cup cooked quinoa
- 1/2 cup diced tomatoes
- 1/4 cup chopped fresh parsley
- 1/4 cup chopped fresh mint
- 1/4 cup chopped red onion
- Juice of 1 lemon
- Salt and pepper to taste

Instructions:
1. Prepare grape leaves according to package instructions if using canned.
2. In a bowl, mix cooked quinoa, diced tomatoes, parsley, mint, red onion, lemon juice, salt, and pepper.
3. Place a spoonful of the quinoa mixture onto each grape leaf and roll it up tightly. Serve chilled.

12. Vegan Stuffed Mushrooms

Ingredients:
- Large button mushrooms, stems removed
- 1 cup cooked quinoa or breadcrumbs
- 1/4 cup chopped onion
- 1/4 cup diced bell peppers
- 2 cloves garlic, minced
- Fresh herbs (such as thyme or rosemary)
- Salt and pepper to taste
- Olive oil for brushing

Instructions:
1. Preheat oven to 375°F (190°C).
2. Mix cooked quinoa or breadcrumbs, chopped onion, diced bell peppers, minced garlic, fresh herbs, salt, and pepper in a bowl.
3. Stuff mushroom caps with the quinoa mixture and place them on a baking sheet.
4. Brush the tops of the mushrooms with olive oil.
5. Bake for 15-20 minutes until mushrooms are tender.

13. Vegan Spinach and Artichoke Phyllo Cups

Ingredients:
- Phyllo pastry cups
- 1 cup chopped spinach, cooked and drained
- 1/2 cup chopped artichoke hearts
- 1/4 cup vegan cream cheese
- 2 tablespoons nutritional yeast
- 1 clove garlic, minced
- Salt and pepper to taste

Instructions:
1. Preheat oven to 350°F (175°C).
2. In a bowl, mix cooked spinach, chopped artichoke hearts, vegan cream cheese, nutritional yeast, minced garlic, salt, and pepper.
3. Spoon the mixture into phyllo pastry cups.
4. Bake for 10-12 minutes until phyllo cups are golden and crispy.

14. Vegan Zucchini Fritters

Ingredients:
- 2 medium zucchinis, grated and squeezed to remove excess moisture
- 1/4 cup chickpea flour
- 2 tablespoons nutritional yeast
- 1 teaspoon baking powder
- 1/2 teaspoon garlic powder

- Salt and pepper to taste
- Oil for frying

Instructions:
1. In a bowl, combine grated zucchini, chickpea flour, nutritional yeast, baking powder, garlic powder, salt, and pepper.
2. Heat oil in a pan over medium heat.
3. Spoon the zucchini mixture into the pan and flatten with a spatula.
4. Cook for 3-4 minutes on each side until golden brown.
5. Drain on paper towels and serve warm.

15. Vegan Cauliflower Wings

Ingredients:
- 1 head cauliflower, cut into florets
- 3/4 cup almond flour or breadcrumbs
- 1 teaspoon garlic powder
- 1 teaspoon onion powder
- 1/2 teaspoon smoked paprika
- Salt and pepper to taste
- 1/2 cup buffalo sauce
  Vegan ranch or blue cheese dressing for dipping

Instructions:
1. Preheat oven to 450°F (230°C). Line a baking sheet with parchment paper.
2. In a bowl, mix almond flour or breadcrumbs, garlic powder, onion powder, smoked paprika, salt, and pepper.
3. Dip cauliflower florets into the mixture and place them on the baking sheet.
4. Bake for 20-25 minutes until crispy and golden brown.
5. Toss the baked cauliflower in buffalo sauce.
6. Serve with vegan ranch or blue cheese dressing for dipping.

16. Vegan Soba Noodle Salad Cups

Ingredients:
- Soba noodles, cooked and cooled
- Rice paper wrappers
- Shredded carrots
- Thinly sliced cucumbers
- Fresh cilantro leaves
- Sesame seeds
- Soy sauce or tamari for dipping

Instructions:
1. Dip a rice paper wrapper in warm water to soften.
2. Lay the wrapper flat and add a small amount of cooked soba noodles, shredded carrots, sliced cucumbers, cilantro leaves, and sesame seeds.
3. Roll the wrapper tightly, tucking in the sides as you go.
4. Serve with soy sauce or tamari for dipping.

17. Vegan Tofu Skewers

Ingredients:
- Extra-firm tofu, pressed and cubed
- Assorted vegetables (bell peppers, onions, cherry tomatoes)
- Marinade: soy sauce or tamari, maple syrup, minced garlic, grated ginger

Instructions:
1. Thread tofu cubes and vegetables onto skewers.
2. Mix the marinade ingredients in a bowl.
3. Brush the marinade over the skewers.
4. Grill or bake the skewers until tofu is lightly browned and vegetables are tender.

18. Vegan Spiced Almonds

Ingredients:
- 2 cups raw almonds
- 1 tablespoon olive oil
- 1 teaspoon ground cumin
- 1 teaspoon smoked paprika
- 1/2 teaspoon cinnamon
- 1/2 teaspoon cayenne pepper (adjust to taste)
- Salt to taste

Instructions:
1. Preheat oven to 300°F (150°C).
2. Toss raw almonds with olive oil, ground cumin, smoked paprika, cinnamon, cayenne pepper, and salt in a bowl.
3. Spread the almonds on a baking sheet.
4. Roast for 20-25 minutes, stirring occasionally, until fragrant and lightly toasted.

19. Vegan Quinoa Stuffed Bell Peppers

Ingredients:
- Mini bell peppers, halved and deseeded
- Cooked quinoa
- Black beans, drained and rinsed
- Diced tomatoes
- Chopped fresh cilantro
- Lime juice
- Salt and pepper to taste

Instructions:
1. Mix cooked quinoa, black beans, diced tomatoes, chopped cilantro, lime juice, salt, and pepper in a bowl.
2. Fill mini bell pepper halves with the quinoa mixture.
3. Serve as stuffed pepper bites.

20. Vegan Edamame Hummus

Ingredients:
- 2 cups shelled edamame, cooked
- 1/4 cup tahini
- Juice of 1 lemon
- 2 cloves garlic, minced
- 2 tablespoons olive oil
- Salt and pepper to taste
- Water (as needed for consistency)

Instructions:
1. Blend cooked edamame, tahini, lemon juice, minced garlic, olive oil, salt, and pepper in a food processor until smooth.
2. Add water as needed for desired consistency.
3. Serve as a dip with vegetable sticks or whole grain crackers.

Chapter 6: Soups

1. Vegan Lentil Soup

Ingredients:
- 1 cup dried red lentils, rinsed
- 4 cups vegetable broth
- 1 onion, diced
- 2 carrots, chopped
- 2 celery stalks, chopped
- 3 cloves garlic, minced
- 1 teaspoon ground cumin
- 1 teaspoon ground turmeric
- 1 teaspoon paprika
- 1 bay leaf
- Salt and pepper to taste
- Fresh cilantro for garnish

Instructions:
1. In a pot, sauté onion, carrots, celery, and garlic until softened.
2. Add lentils, vegetable broth, cumin, turmeric, paprika, bay leaf, salt, and pepper. Stir well.
3. Bring to a boil, then reduce heat, cover, and simmer for 20-25 minutes until lentils are tender.
4. Remove the bay leaf, blend part of the soup for a creamier texture if desired.
5. Serve garnished with fresh cilantro.

2. Vegan Butternut Squash Soup

Ingredients:
- 1 butternut squash, peeled, seeded, and cubed
- 1 onion, diced
- 2 cloves garlic, minced
- 4 cups vegetable broth

- 1 teaspoon ground cinnamon
- 1/2 teaspoon ground nutmeg
- 1/4 teaspoon cayenne pepper (optional)
- Salt and pepper to taste
- Coconut cream for garnish

Instructions:
1. In a pot, sauté onion and garlic until translucent.
2. Add cubed butternut squash, vegetable broth, cinnamon, nutmeg, cayenne pepper, salt, and pepper. Stir well.
3. Bring to a boil, then reduce heat and simmer for 20-25 minutes until squash is tender.
4. Blend the soup until smooth using an immersion blender or regular blender.
5. Serve with a swirl of coconut cream on top.

3. Vegan Tomato Basil Soup

Ingredients:
- 6 tomatoes, chopped
- 1 onion, diced
- 3 cloves garlic, minced
- 4 cups vegetable broth
- 1/4 cup fresh basil leaves
- 2 tablespoons tomato paste
- 1 teaspoon dried oregano
- Salt and pepper to taste
- Olive oil for sautéing
- Fresh basil for garnish

Instructions:
1. In a pot, sauté onion and garlic in olive oil until softened.
2. Add chopped tomatoes, vegetable broth, basil leaves, tomato paste, dried oregano, salt, and pepper. Stir well.
3. Bring to a boil, then reduce heat and simmer for 20-25 minutes.

4. Blend the soup until smooth using an immersion blender or regular blender.
5. Serve garnished with fresh basil.

4. Vegan Miso Soup

Ingredients:
- 4 cups vegetable broth
- 2 tablespoons miso paste
- 1 block firm tofu, cubed
- 1 cup sliced shiitake mushrooms
- 2 green onions, chopped
- 1 sheet nori seaweed, torn into pieces
- 1 tablespoon soy sauce or tamari
- 1 teaspoon sesame oil (optional)

Instructions:
1. In a pot, bring vegetable broth to a simmer.
2. In a small bowl, dissolve miso paste in a little warm water and add it to the broth.
3. Add cubed tofu, sliced mushrooms, green onions, torn nori, soy sauce, and sesame oil to the pot.
4. Simmer for 5-7 minutes until heated through.
5. Serve hot.

5. Vegan Coconut Curry Soup

Ingredients:
- 1 tablespoon coconut oil
- 1 onion, diced
- 2 cloves garlic, minced
- 2 tablespoons red curry paste
- 1 can (14 oz) coconut milk
- 4 cups vegetable broth
- 2 cups diced sweet potatoes

- 1 cup chopped kale or spinach
- 1 tablespoon lime juice
- Salt and pepper to taste
- Fresh cilantro for garnish

Instructions:
1. In a pot, sauté onion and garlic in coconut oil until fragrant.
2. Stir in red curry paste and cook for 1-2 minutes.
3. Add coconut milk, vegetable broth, diced sweet potatoes, salt, and pepper. Bring to a boil, then simmer for 15-20 minutes until sweet potatoes are tender.
4. Stir in chopped kale or spinach and lime juice. Cook for an additional 5 minutes.
5. Serve garnished with fresh cilantro.

 6. Vegan Potato Leek Soup

Ingredients:
- 3 leeks, sliced (white and light green parts only)
- 3 potatoes, peeled and diced
- 4 cups vegetable broth
- 1 cup unsweetened almond milk
- 2 tablespoons nutritional yeast
- 1 bay leaf
- Salt and pepper to taste
- Chopped chives for garnish

Instructions:
1. In a pot, sauté sliced leeks until softened.
2. Add diced potatoes, vegetable broth, almond milk, nutritional yeast, bay leaf, salt, and pepper. Bring to a boil, then reduce heat and simmer for 20-25 minutes until potatoes are tender.
3. Remove the bay leaf, blend part of the soup for creaminess if desired.
4. Serve hot, garnished with chopped chives.

7. Vegan Spicy Black Bean Soup

Ingredients:
- 2 cans (15 oz each) black beans, drained and rinsed
- 1 onion, diced
- 2 cloves garlic, minced
- 1 red bell pepper, diced
- 4 cups vegetable broth
- 1 teaspoon ground cumin
- 1 teaspoon chili powder
- 1/2 teaspoon smoked paprika
- Juice of 1 lime
- Salt and pepper to taste
- Fresh cilantro for garnish

Instructions:
1. In a pot, sauté onion, garlic, and red bell pepper until softened.
2. Add black beans, vegetable broth, ground cumin, chili powder, smoked paprika, salt, and pepper. Stir well.
3. Simmer for 15-20 minutes to allow flavors to meld.
4. Stir in lime juice.
5. Serve hot, garnished with fresh cilantro.

8. Vegan Minestrone Soup

Ingredients:
- 1 onion, diced
- 2 carrots, chopped
- 2 celery stalks, chopped
- 3 cloves garlic, minced
- 1 can (15 oz) diced tomatoes
- 6 cups vegetable broth
- 1 cup cooked small pasta (like ditalini or elbow macaroni)
- 1 can (15 oz) kidney beans, drained and rinsed
- 1 teaspoon dried basil

- 1 teaspoon dried oregano
- Salt and pepper to taste
- Fresh parsley for garnish

Instructions:
1. In a pot, sauté onion, carrots, celery, and garlic until softened.
2. Add diced tomatoes, vegetable broth, cooked pasta, kidney beans, dried basil, dried oregano, salt, and pepper. Stir well.
3. Simmer for 15-20 minutes.
4. Serve hot, garnished with fresh parsley.

9. Vegan Thai Coconut Soup (Tom Kha)

Ingredients:
- 4 cups vegetable broth
- 1 can (14 oz) coconut milk
- 1 lemongrass stalk, smashed
- 3 kaffir lime leaves
- 2-inch piece of galangal or ginger, sliced
- 1 cup sliced mushrooms
- 1 red chili, sliced
- 1 tablespoon soy sauce or tamari
- 1 tablespoon lime juice
- Fresh cilantro for garnish

Instructions:
1. In a pot, bring vegetable broth and coconut milk to a simmer.
2. Add smashed lemongrass stalk, kaffir lime leaves, sliced galangal or ginger, sliced mushrooms, sliced red chili, soy sauce or tamari, and lime juice.
3. Simmer for 10-15 minutes.
4. Remove lemongrass, kaffir lime leaves, and galangal or ginger slices before serving.
5. Serve hot, garnished with fresh cilantro.

10. Vegan Broccoli Soup

Ingredients:
- 1 onion, diced
- 3 cups chopped broccoli florets
- 4 cups vegetable broth
- 1 cup unsweetened almond milk
- 2 tablespoons nutritional yeast
- 2 tablespoons tahini
- 2 cloves garlic, minced
- Salt and pepper to taste
- Olive oil for sautéing

Instructions:
1. In a pot, sauté onion and minced garlic in olive oil until translucent.
2. Add chopped broccoli florets, vegetable broth, almond milk, nutritional yeast, tahini, salt, and pepper. Bring to a boil, then reduce heat and simmer for 15-20 minutes until broccoli is tender.
3. Blend the soup until smooth using an immersion blender or regular blender.
4. Serve hot.

11. Vegan Carrot Ginger Soup

Ingredients:
- 6 carrots, peeled and chopped
- 1 onion, diced
- 2 cloves garlic, minced
- 2 tablespoons fresh ginger, grated
- 4 cups vegetable broth
- 1 can (14 oz) coconut milk
- 1 tablespoon olive oil
- Salt and pepper to taste
- Fresh cilantro or parsley for garnish

Instructions:
1. In a pot, sauté onion, garlic, and grated ginger in olive oil until fragrant.
2. Add chopped carrots and vegetable broth. Bring to a boil, then reduce heat and simmer for 15-20 minutes until carrots are tender.
3. Blend the soup until smooth using an immersion blender or regular blender.
4. Stir in coconut milk and simmer for an additional 5 minutes.
5. Season with salt and pepper.
6. Serve hot, garnished with fresh cilantro or parsley.

12. Vegan Corn Chowder

Ingredients:
- 4 cups corn kernels (fresh or frozen)
- 1 onion, diced
- 2 cloves garlic, minced
- 3 potatoes, peeled and diced
- 4 cups vegetable broth
- 1 cup unsweetened almond milk
- 2 tablespoons nutritional yeast
- 1 teaspoon smoked paprika
- Salt and pepper to taste
- Fresh chives for garnish

Instructions:
1. In a pot, sauté onion and garlic until translucent.
2. Add corn kernels, diced potatoes, and vegetable broth. Bring to a boil, then simmer for 15-20 minutes until potatoes are cooked.
3. Blend part of the soup for creaminess if desired.
4. Stir in almond milk, nutritional yeast, smoked paprika, salt, and pepper.
5. Simmer for an additional 5 minutes.
6. Serve hot, garnished with fresh chives.

13. Vegan Beetroot Soup (Borscht)

Ingredients:
- 3 beetroots, peeled and grated
- 1 onion, diced
- 2 carrots, grated
- 4 cups vegetable broth
- 2 tablespoons apple cider vinegar
- 1 bay leaf
- Salt and pepper to taste
- Vegan sour cream or coconut yogurt for garnish
- Fresh dill for garnish

Instructions:
1. In a pot, sauté onion until translucent.
2. Add grated beetroots, grated carrots, vegetable broth, apple cider vinegar, bay leaf, salt, and pepper. Simmer for 25-30 minutes until vegetables are tender.
3. Remove the bay leaf, blend part of the soup for a smoother consistency if desired.
4. Serve hot, garnished with a dollop of vegan sour cream or coconut yogurt and fresh dill.

14. Vegan Mushroom Barley Soup

Ingredients:
- 1 cup pearl barley, rinsed
- 2 tablespoons olive oil
- 1 onion, diced
- 3 cloves garlic, minced
- 8 oz mushrooms, sliced
- 4 cups vegetable broth
- 1 teaspoon dried thyme
- Salt and pepper to taste
- Fresh parsley for garnish

Instructions:
1. In a pot, heat olive oil and sauté onion and garlic until softened.
2. Add sliced mushrooms and cook until they release their moisture.
3. Stir in pearl barley, vegetable broth, dried thyme, salt, and pepper. Bring to a boil, then reduce heat and simmer for 30-35 minutes until barley is tender.
4. Serve hot, garnished with fresh parsley.

15. Vegan Asparagus Soup

Ingredients:
- 1 bunch asparagus, trimmed and chopped
- 1 onion, diced
- 2 cloves garlic, minced
- 4 cups vegetable broth
- 1 potato, peeled and diced
- 1/2 cup unsweetened coconut milk
- 1 tablespoon lemon juice
- Salt and pepper to taste
- Lemon zest for garnish

Instructions:
1. In a pot, sauté onion and garlic until translucent.
2. Add chopped asparagus, diced potato, and vegetable broth. Bring to a boil, then simmer for 15-20 minutes until vegetables are tender.
3. Blend the soup until smooth using an immersion blender or regular blender.
4. Stir in coconut milk and lemon juice.
5. Season with salt and pepper.
6. Serve hot, garnished with lemon zest.

16. Vegan Pumpkin Soup

Ingredients:
- 2 cups pumpkin puree (canned or homemade)
- 1 onion, diced
- 2 cloves garlic, minced
- 4 cups vegetable broth
- 1 can (14 oz) coconut milk
- 1 teaspoon ground cumin
- 1/2 teaspoon ground cinnamon
- Salt and pepper to taste
- Pepitas (pumpkin seeds) for garnish

Instructions:
1. In a pot, sauté onion and garlic until softened.
2. Add pumpkin puree, vegetable broth, coconut milk, ground cumin, ground cinnamon, salt, and pepper. Stir well.
3. Bring to a simmer and cook for 10-15 minutes.
4. Serve hot, garnished with pepitas.

17. Vegan Spinach Soup

Ingredients:
- 6 cups fresh spinach leaves
- 1 onion, diced
- 2 cloves garlic, minced
- 4 cups vegetable broth
- 1 potato, peeled and diced
- 1/2 cup unsweetened almond milk
- 1 tablespoon nutritional yeast
- Salt and pepper to taste
- Nutmeg for garnish

Instructions:
1. In a pot, sauté onion and garlic until translucent.

2. Add fresh spinach leaves, diced potato, and vegetable broth. Simmer for 10-12 minutes until potatoes are tender.
3. Blend the soup until smooth using an immersion blender or regular blender.
4. Stir in almond milk, nutritional yeast, salt, and pepper.
5. Season with a sprinkle of nutmeg.
6. Serve hot.

18. Vegan Red Lentil Soup with Coconut

Ingredients:
- 1 cup red lentils, rinsed
- 1 onion, diced
- 2 cloves garlic, minced
- 1 can (14 oz) diced tomatoes
- 4 cups vegetable broth
- 1 can (14 oz) coconut milk
- 1 teaspoon ground turmeric
- 1 teaspoon ground cumin
- Salt and pepper to taste
- Fresh cilantro for garnish

Instructions:
1. In a pot, sauté onion and garlic until fragrant.
2. Add red lentils, diced tomatoes, vegetable broth, coconut milk, ground turmeric, ground cumin, salt, and pepper. Stir well.
3. Bring to a boil, then reduce heat and simmer for 20-25 minutes until lentils are cooked.
4. Serve hot, garnished with fresh cilantro.

19. Vegan Lemon Rice Soup (Avgolemono)

Ingredients:
- 1 cup cooked rice
- 4 cups vegetable broth

- Juice of 2 lemons
- Zest of 1 lemon
- 2 tablespoons cornstarch
- 1 onion, diced
- 2 cloves garlic, minced
- Salt and pepper to taste
- Fresh dill for garnish

Instructions:
1. In a pot, sauté onion and garlic until softened.
2. Add vegetable broth and bring to a simmer.
3. In a small bowl, whisk together lemon juice, lemon zest, and cornstarch. Add it to the simmering broth while stirring continuously until slightly thickened.
4. Stir in cooked rice and simmer for a few minutes.
5. Season with salt and pepper.
6. Serve hot, garnished with fresh dill.

20. Vegan Spiced Cauliflower Soup

Ingredients:
- 1 head cauliflower, chopped
- 1 onion, diced
- 2 cloves garlic, minced
- 4 cups vegetable broth
- 1 can (14 oz) coconut milk
- 1 teaspoon ground coriander
- 1/2 teaspoon ground turmeric
- 1/2 teaspoon smoked paprika
- Salt and pepper to taste
- Toasted almonds for garnish

Instructions:
1. In a pot, sauté onion and garlic until translucent.

2. Add chopped cauliflower, vegetable broth, coconut milk, ground coriander, ground turmeric, smoked paprika, salt, and pepper. Stir well.

3. Bring to a boil, then reduce heat and simmer for 20-25 minutes until cauliflower is tender.

4. Blend the soup until smooth using an immersion blender or regular blender.

5. Serve hot, garnished with toasted almonds.

Chapter 7: Herbal Teas and Elixirs

1. Turmeric Ginger Tea

Ingredients:
- 1-inch piece of fresh turmeric root, sliced
- 1-inch piece of fresh ginger, sliced
- 4 cups water
- Lemon wedges (optional)
- Raw honey or maple syrup (optional)

Instructions:
1. In a saucepan, bring water to a boil.
2. Add turmeric and ginger slices to the boiling water.
3. Simmer for 10-15 minutes.
4. Strain the tea into cups.
5. Optionally, add a squeeze of lemon juice and sweeten with raw honey or maple syrup to taste.

2. Cinnamon Cardamom Tea

Ingredients:
- 2 cinnamon sticks
- 4-5 green cardamom pods, lightly crushed
- 4 cups water
- Plant-based milk (optional)
- Sweetener of choice (optional)

Instructions:
1. In a pot, bring water to a boil.
2. Add cinnamon sticks and crushed cardamom pods to the boiling water.
3. Simmer for 10-15 minutes.
4. Strain the tea into cups.
5. Optionally, add a splash of plant-based milk and sweeten with your preferred sweetener.

3. Ashwagandha Elixir

Ingredients:
- 1 teaspoon ashwagandha powder
- 1 teaspoon maca powder
- 1 teaspoon raw cacao powder
- 1 cup warm plant-based milk (almond, coconut, or oat)
- 1 teaspoon coconut oil
- Raw honey or maple syrup (optional)

Instructions:
1. In a mug, mix ashwagandha, maca, and raw cacao powders.
2. Pour warm plant-based milk into the mug.
3. Add coconut oil and stir until well combined.
4. Optionally, sweeten with raw honey or maple syrup to taste.

4. Holy Basil (Tulsi) Adaptogenic Elixir

Ingredients:
- 1 tablespoon dried holy basil (Tulsi) leaves
- 1 teaspoon dried rose petals (optional)
- 2 cups water
- 1 teaspoon honey (optional)

Instructions:
1. In a saucepan, bring water to a boil.
2. Add dried holy basil leaves and rose petals (if using) to the boiling water.
3. Simmer for 10-15 minutes.
4. Strain the elixir into cups.
5. Optionally, sweeten with honey.

5. Licorice Fennel Digestive Elixir

Ingredients:
- 1 teaspoon licorice root

- 1 teaspoon fennel seeds
- 2 cups water
- Fresh lemon slices (optional)

Instructions:
1. In a saucepan, bring water to a boil.
2. Add licorice root and fennel seeds to the boiling water.
3. Simmer for 10-15 minutes.
4. Strain the elixir into cups.
5. Optionally, add fresh lemon slices for flavor.

6. Chamomile Lavender Tea

Ingredients:
- 2 teaspoons dried chamomile flowers
- 1 teaspoon dried lavender buds
- 2 cups hot water
- Raw honey (optional)

Instructions:
1. Place chamomile flowers and lavender buds in a teapot or infuser.
2. Pour hot water over the herbs and let steep for 5-7 minutes.
3. Strain the tea into cups.
4. Optionally, sweeten with raw honey if desired.

7. Peppermint Licorice Tea

Ingredients:
- 1 tablespoon dried peppermint leaves
- 1 teaspoon licorice root
- 2 cups hot water
- Fresh mint leaves for garnish (optional)

Instructions:
1. Combine dried peppermint leaves and licorice root in a teapot or infuser.

2. Pour hot water over the herbs and let steep for 5-7 minutes.
3. Strain the tea into cups.
4. Garnish with fresh mint leaves if desired.

8. Triphala Detox Elixir

Ingredients:
- 1 teaspoon Triphala powder
- 1 teaspoon fresh lemon juice
- 1 teaspoon raw honey
- 1 cup warm water

Instructions:
1. Mix Triphala powder with warm water.
2. Add fresh lemon juice and raw honey.
3. Stir well until thoroughly combined.
4. Consume this elixir in the morning on an empty stomach for detoxification.

9. Brahmi Gotu Kola Brain Tonic

Ingredients:
- 1 teaspoon dried Brahmi (Bacopa) leaves
- 1 teaspoon dried Gotu Kola leaves
- 2 cups hot water
- 1 teaspoon coconut oil (optional)

Instructions:
1. Steep dried Brahmi and Gotu Kola leaves in hot water for 10-15 minutes.
2. Strain the herbal infusion into cups.
3. Optionally, add a teaspoon of coconut oil for an added brain boost.

10. Rose Hibiscus Elixir

Ingredients:
- 1 tablespoon dried hibiscus flowers
- 1 tablespoon dried rose petals
- 2 cups hot water
- Fresh rose petals for garnish (optional)

Instructions:
1. Steep dried hibiscus flowers and rose petals in hot water for 5-7 minutes.
2. Strain the elixir into cups.
3. Garnish with fresh rose petals for an elegant touch.

11. Ginger Lemon Detox Elixir

Ingredients:
- 1-inch piece fresh ginger, thinly sliced
- Juice of 1 lemon
- 2 cups hot water
- Raw honey (optional)

Instructions:
1. Steep fresh ginger slices in hot water for 5-10 minutes.
2. Squeeze in the juice of one lemon.
3. Optionally, sweeten with raw honey to taste.

12. Dandelion Burdock Cleansing Elixir

Ingredients:
- 1 tablespoon dried dandelion root
- 1 tablespoon dried burdock root
- 2 cups hot water
- Fresh lemon slices (optional)

Instructions:
1. Steep dried dandelion root and burdock root in hot water for 10-15 minutes.
2. Strain the elixir into cups.
3. Optionally, add fresh lemon slices for a refreshing twist.

13. Saffron Cardamom Elixir

Ingredients:
- A few strands of saffron
- 2-3 cardamom pods, lightly crushed
- 2 cups hot water
- Coconut milk (optional)
- Sweetener of choice (optional)

Instructions:
1. Steep saffron strands and crushed cardamom pods in hot water for 5-7 minutes.
2. Optionally, add a splash of coconut milk and sweeten to taste.

14. Astragalus Elderberry Immune Elixir

Ingredients:
- 1 teaspoon dried astragalus root
- 1 tablespoon dried elderberries
- 2 cups hot water
- Raw honey (optional)

Instructions:
1. Steep dried astragalus root and elderberries in hot water for 10-15 minutes.
2. Strain the elixir into cups.
3. Optionally, sweeten with raw honey for added taste.

15. Lavender Lemon Balm Relaxation Elixir

Ingredients:
- 1 tablespoon dried lavender flowers
- 1 tablespoon dried lemon balm leaves
- 2 cups hot water
- Fresh lemon slices (optional)

Instructions:
1. Steep dried lavender flowers and lemon balm leaves in hot water for 5-7 minutes.
2. Strain the elixir into cups.
3. Optionally, garnish with fresh lemon slices.

16. Lemon Verbena Tea

Ingredients:
- 1 tablespoon dried lemon verbena leaves
- 2 cups hot water
- Lemon slices for garnish (optional)
- Raw honey (optional)

Instructions:
1. Steep dried lemon verbena leaves in hot water for 5-7 minutes.
2. Strain the tea into cups.
3. Garnish with lemon slices if desired.
4. Optionally, sweeten with raw honey to taste.

17. Holy Basil (Tulsi) Rose Tea

Ingredients:
- 1 tablespoon dried holy basil (Tulsi) leaves
- 1 tablespoon dried rose petals
- 2 cups hot water
- Fresh rose petals for garnish (optional)

Instructions:
1. Steep dried holy basil leaves and rose petals in hot water for 5-7 minutes.
2. Strain the tea into cups.
3. Garnish with fresh rose petals for a lovely touch.

18. Schisandra Berry Adaptogenic Elixir

Ingredients:
- 1 teaspoon dried schisandra berries
- 2 cups hot water
- Fresh mint leaves for garnish (optional)
- Raw honey (optional)

Instructions:
1. Steep dried schisandra berries in hot water for 10-15 minutes.
2. Strain the elixir into cups.
3. Garnish with fresh mint leaves if desired.
4. Optionally, sweeten with raw honey.

19. Moringa Ginger Immune Boosting Elixir

Ingredients:
- 1 teaspoon moringa powder
- 1-inch piece fresh ginger, grated
- 2 cups hot water
- Fresh lemon slices (optional)
- Raw honey (optional)

Instructions:
1. Mix moringa powder and grated ginger in hot water.
2. Allow it to steep for 5-7 minutes.
3. Strain the elixir into cups.
4. Optionally, garnish with fresh lemon slices and sweeten with raw honey.

20. Butterfly Pea Flower Blue Tea

Ingredients:
- 1 tablespoon dried butterfly pea flowers
- 2 cups hot water
- Lemon wedges (optional)
- Raw honey or agave syrup (optional)

Instructions:
1. Steep dried butterfly pea flowers in hot water for 5-7 minutes.
2. Strain the tea into cups.
3. Add lemon wedges for color change (turns purple).
4. Optionally, sweeten with raw honey or agave syrup.

Conclusion

Embracing Ayurveda for Long-Term Well-being

In the journey towards holistic health and well-being, the ancient wisdom of Ayurveda serves as a guiding light, offering profound insights and practices to nurture our bodies, minds, and spirits. As we immerse ourselves in the principles of this time-honored system, we unearth not just a means of healing but a philosophy that celebrates harmony and balance in every facet of life.

Holistic Balance: Ayurveda, the science of life, stands as a testament to the profound connection between oneself and the universe. It doesn't merely advocate for physical health but emphasizes the significance of maintaining equilibrium within our unique constitution, allowing us to thrive in a state of balance.

Mindful Living: The beauty of Ayurveda transcends the realms of diet and herbal remedies; it extends to encompass mindfulness, meditation, and lifestyle choices. Encouraging us to sync our daily routines with the rhythms of nature, Ayurveda invites us to awaken to the subtle nuances of our bodies and surroundings.

Personalized Wellness: One of Ayurveda's greatest gifts lies in its recognition of individuality. By acknowledging our distinct doshas, or constitutions, we can tailor lifestyle, diet, and self-care practices to suit our specific needs, promoting a sense of equilibrium and vitality.

Nourishing Nutrition: The Ayurvedic diet, rich in whole foods, herbs, and spices, not only sustains but also heals. Through mindful eating and selecting foods that resonate with our constitution, we unlock the potential for optimal digestion, improved immunity, and sustained energy levels.

Harmony and Wholeness: As we weave Ayurveda's principles into the fabric of our lives, we uncover a path towards greater harmony and wholeness. It's a journey that intertwines the physical, mental, and spiritual aspects of our existence, guiding us towards an enriched and balanced way of being.

In adopting an Ayurvedic lifestyle, we embrace not just a healing modality but a philosophy that encourages us to re-establish a profound connection with ourselves and the world around us. As we honor our bodies, nurture our minds, and listen to the whispers of our spirits, we pave the way for enduring health, vitality, and a profound sense of well-being.

May the timeless wisdom of Ayurveda be a beacon, guiding us towards a life of balance, wellness, and harmony.